Where Did They Go?
Written by Shaleea Venney, PhD
Copyright © 2025 by Shaleea Venney
All rights reserved.

No part of this publication may be reproduced, distributed, or transmitted in any form or by any means, including photocopying, recording, or other electronic or mechanical methods, without the prior written permission of the publisher, except in the case of brief quotations embodied in critical reviews and certain other noncommercial uses permitted by copyright law.

For permission requests, please contact:
After Goodbye
www.aftergoodbyebook.com
support@aftergoodbyebook.com
Printed in the United States of America.
ISBN: 979-8-218-67298-0
First Edition, 2025

For every child who has ever wondered where someone they love has gone…

And for the grown-ups who hold their tiny hands through loss, with courage in their voice and love in their hearts. You are not alone.

— With all my heart,
Shaleea Venney PhD.

Where Did They Go?

A gentle story to help little hearts understand big goodbyes

By
Shaleea Venney, PhD

I looked for you in this morning's light,
But you were gone—just out of sight.

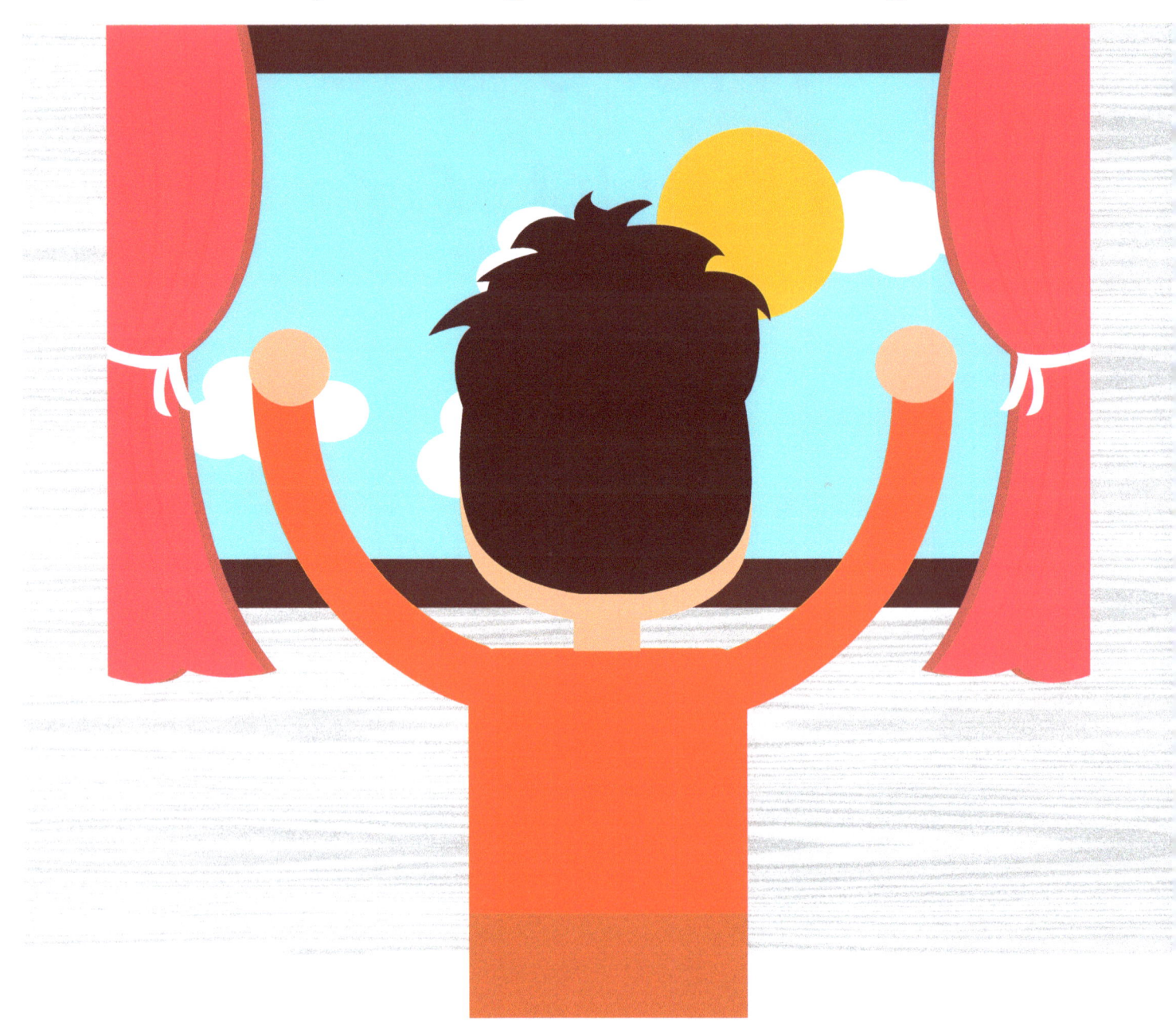

They say you're not here anymore...
But where'd you go? What was it for?

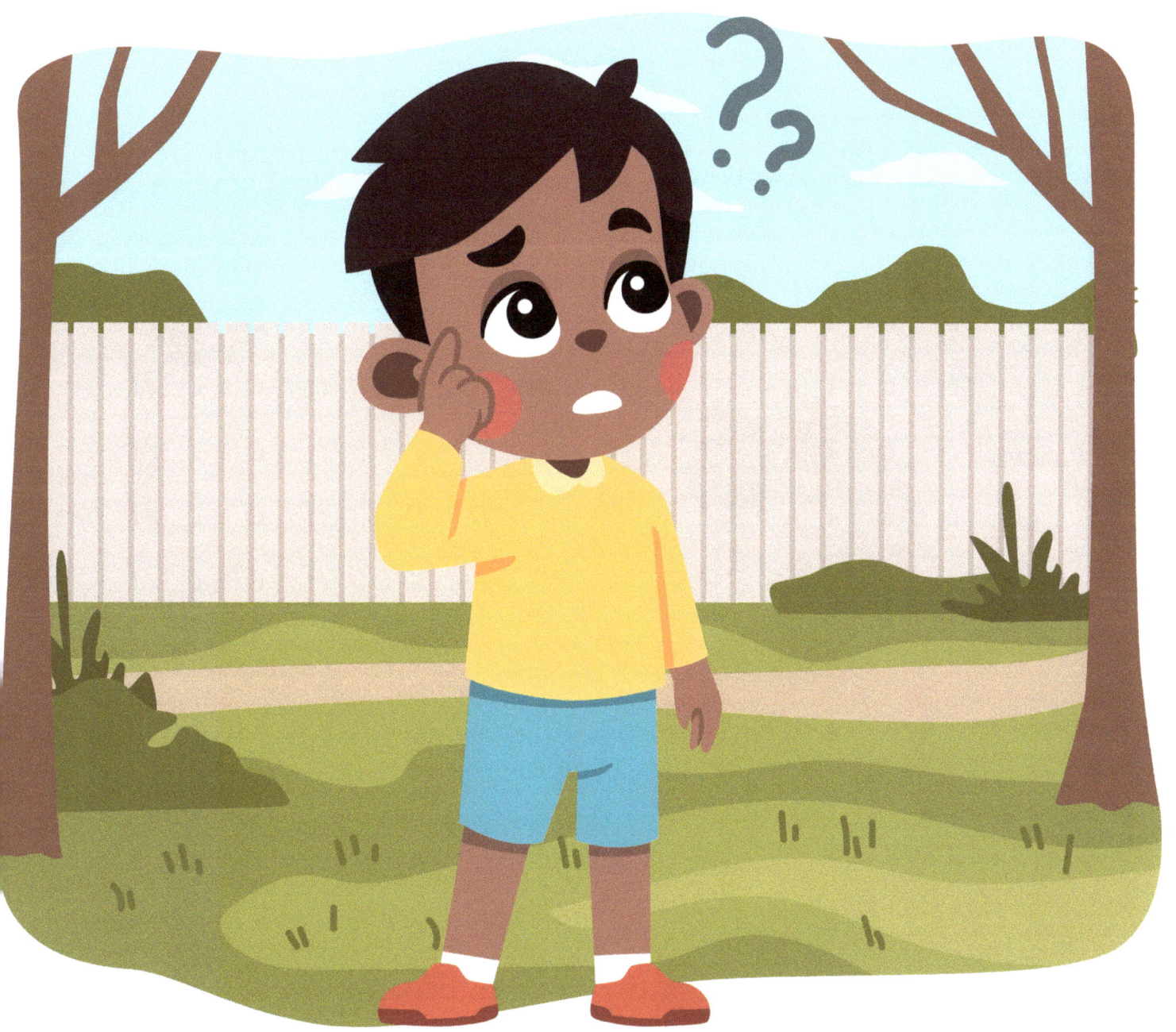

Are you the wind that hugs my face?
The whisper floating through the place?

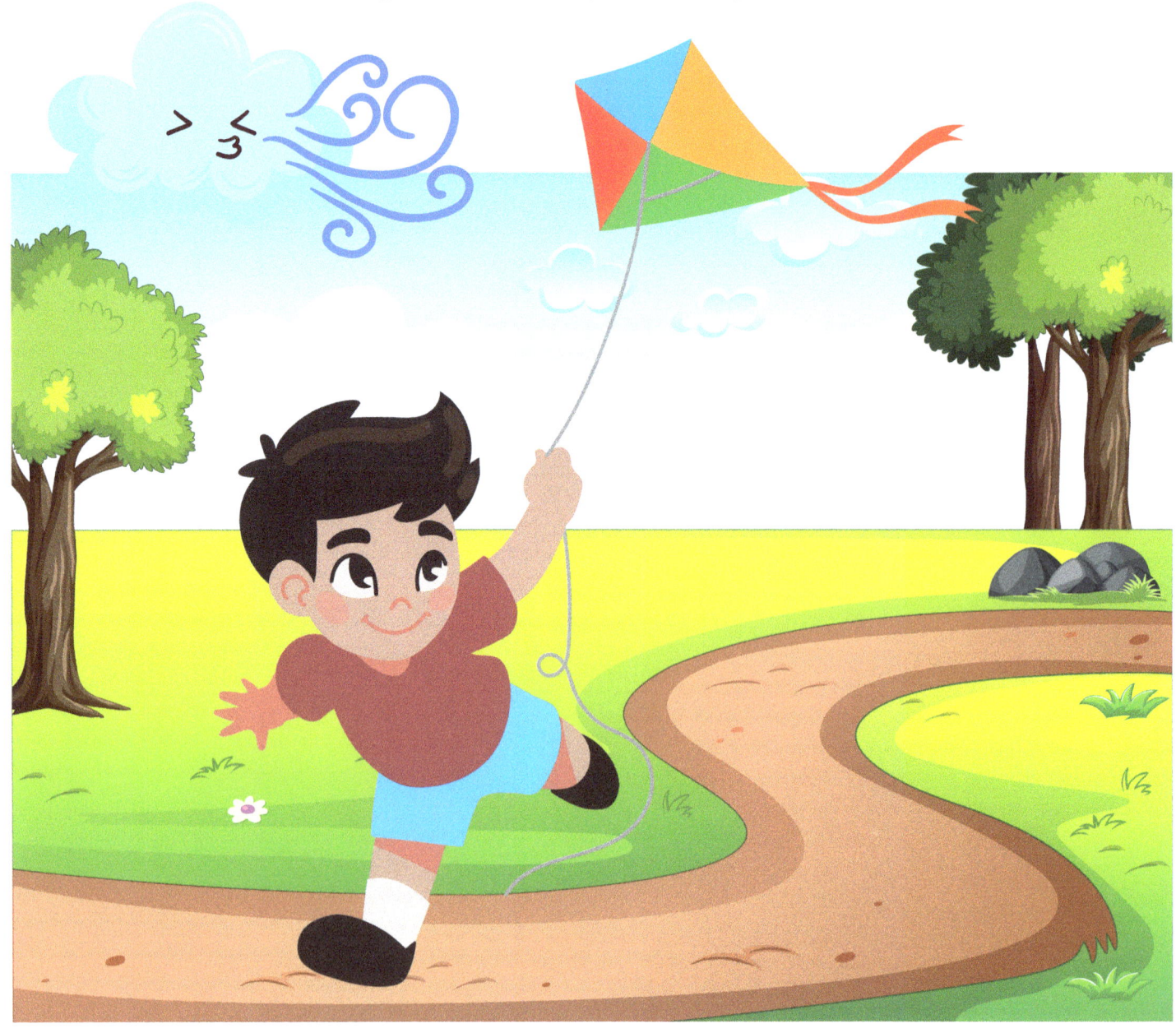

Are you a star up in the sky—
The kind that twinkles when I cry?

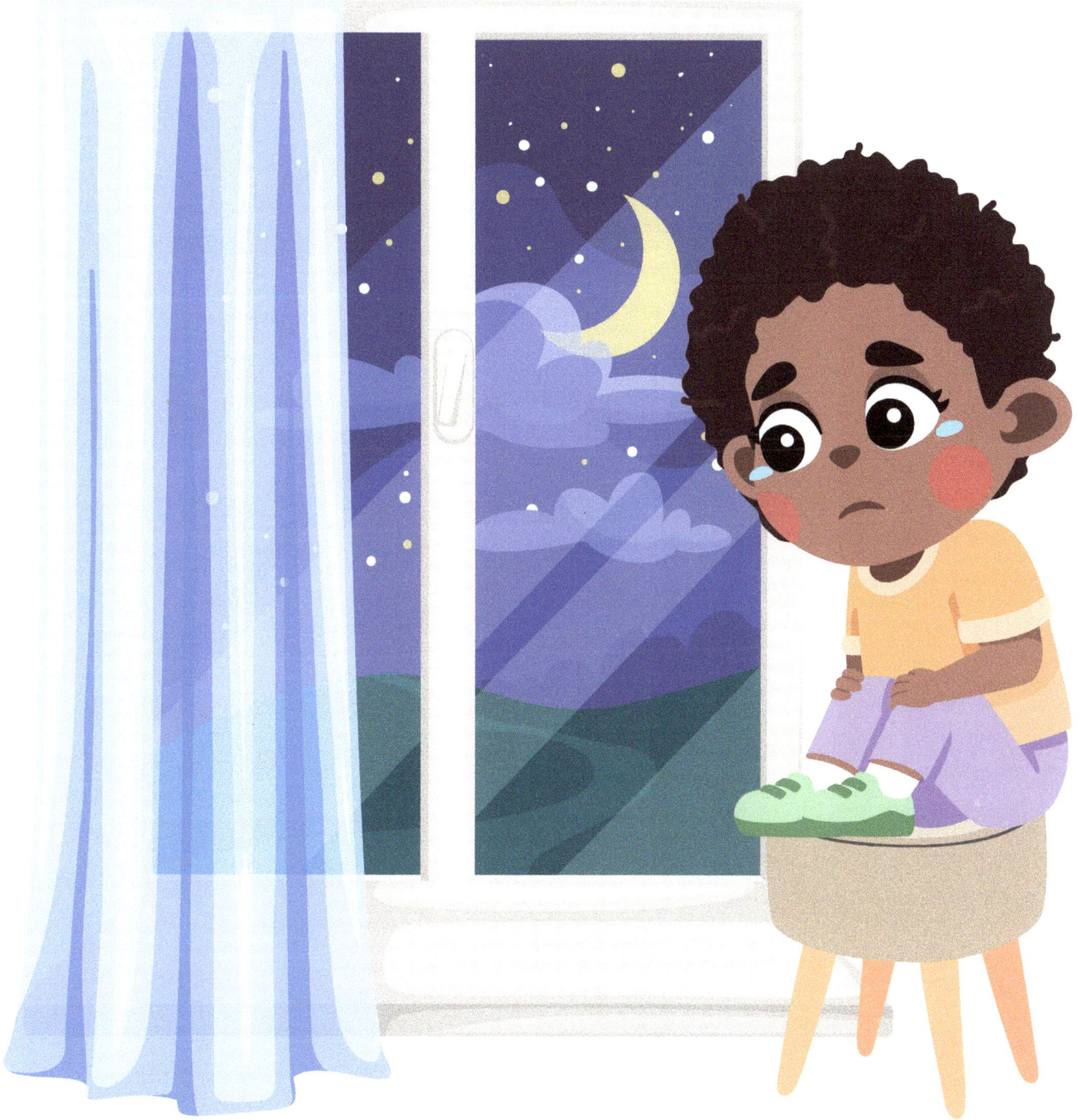

They said your body had to rest—
It tried its hardest, did its best

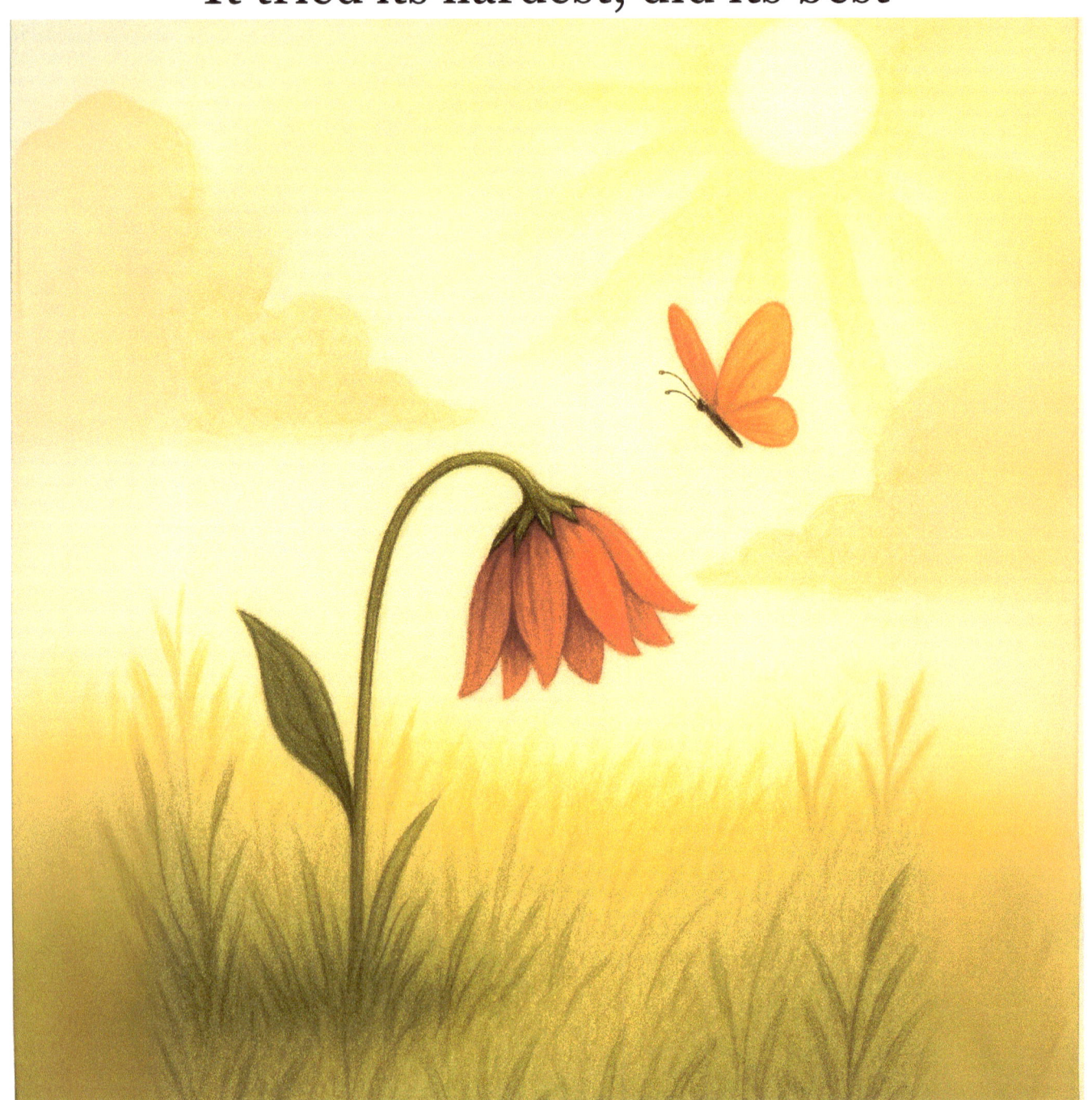

But when a body breaks inside,
It means it's time to say goodbye.

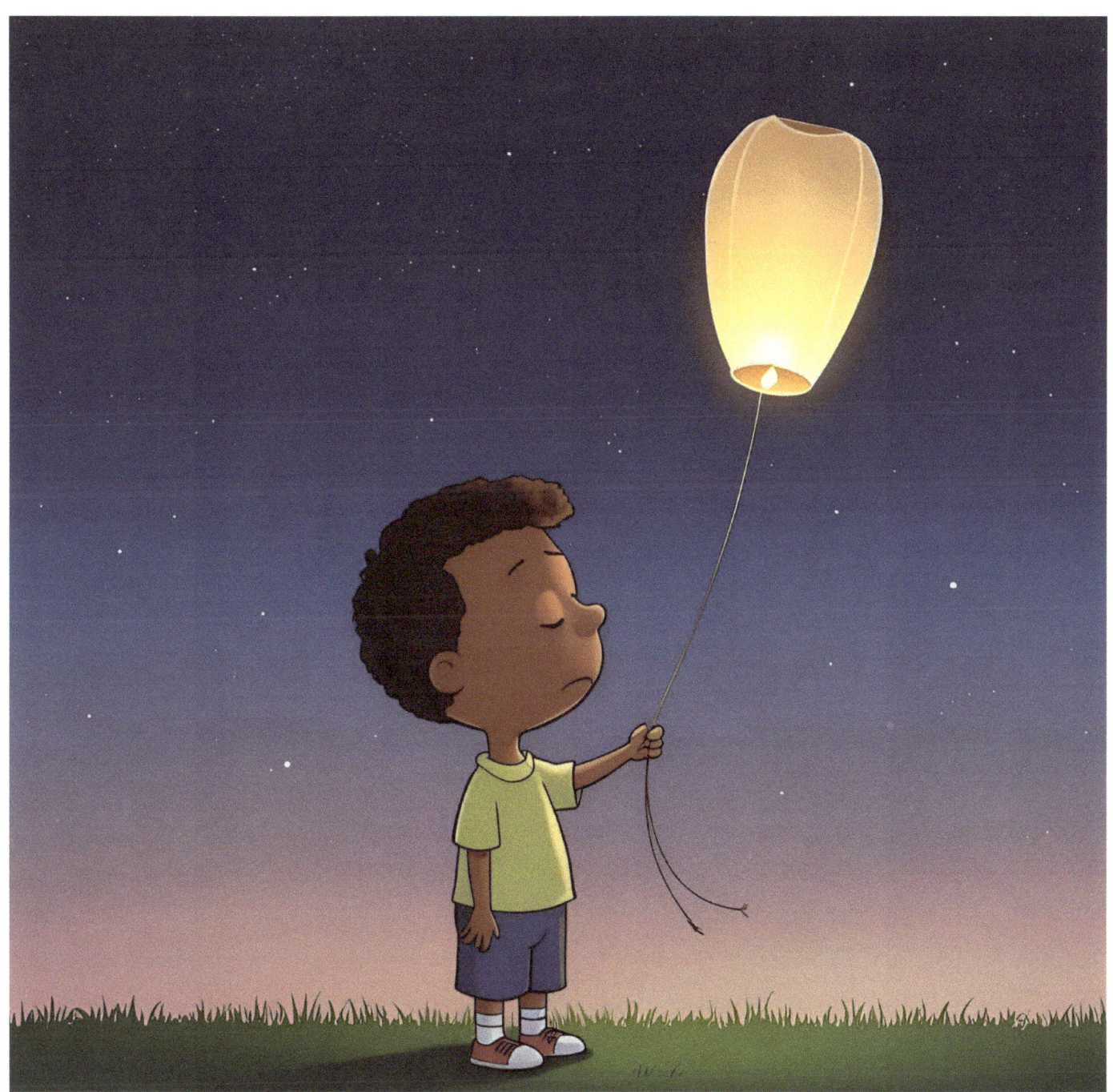

You don't eat snacks or brush your hair.
You're not in bed or your old chair.

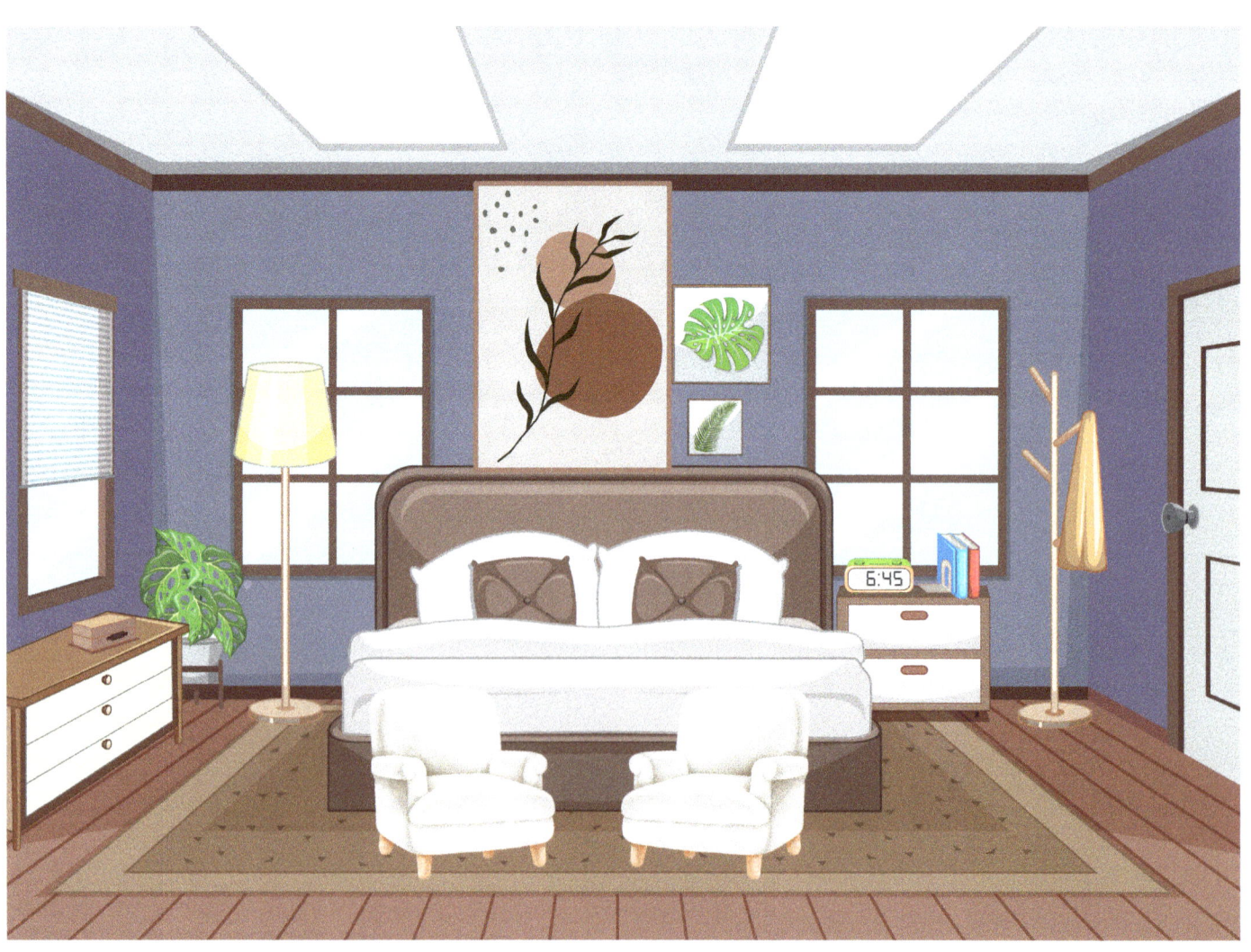

But somehow, when I close my eyes,
I feel you with me, right nearby.

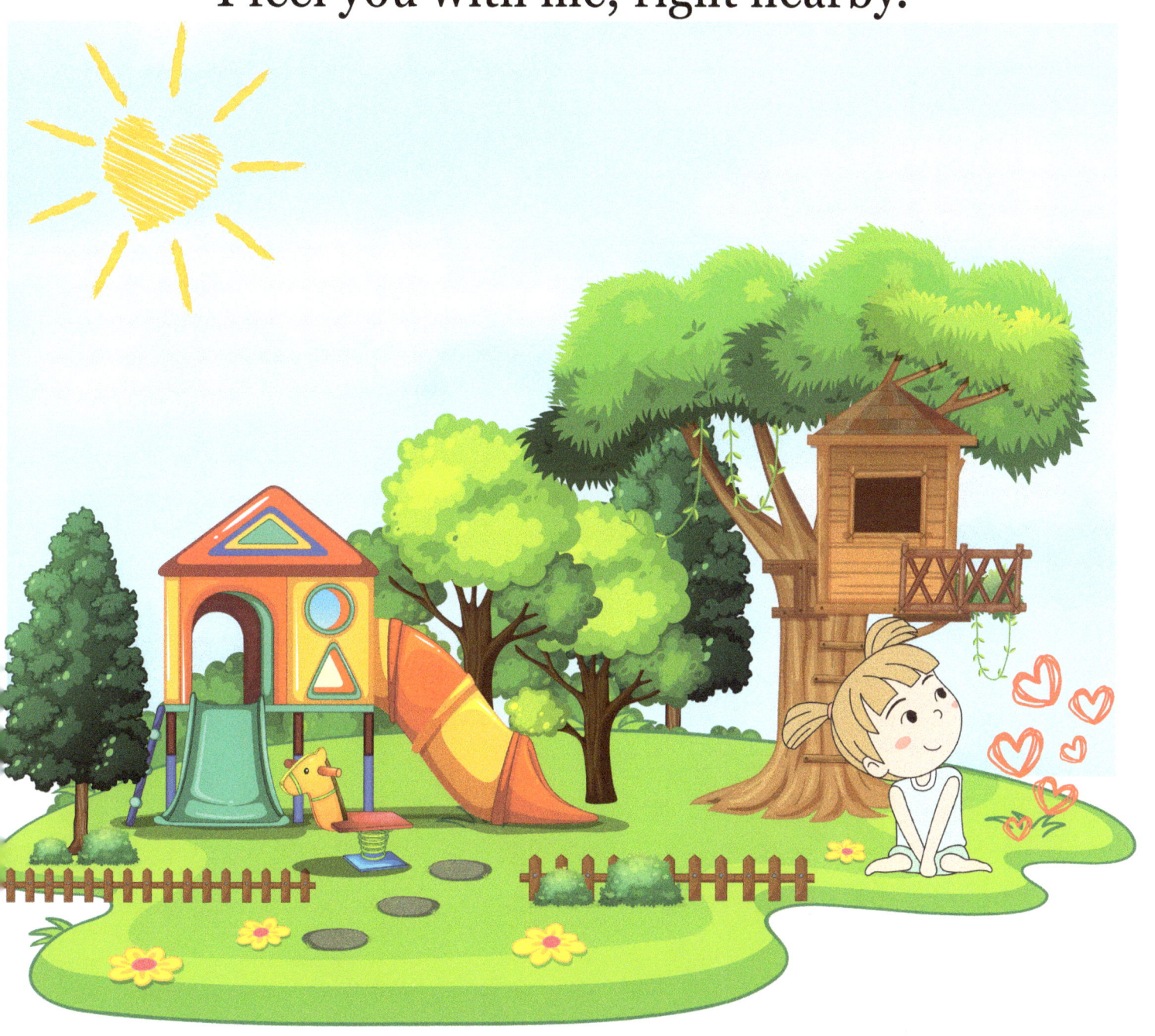

You're in the stories that I know,
The songs you sang, the seeds you'd sow.

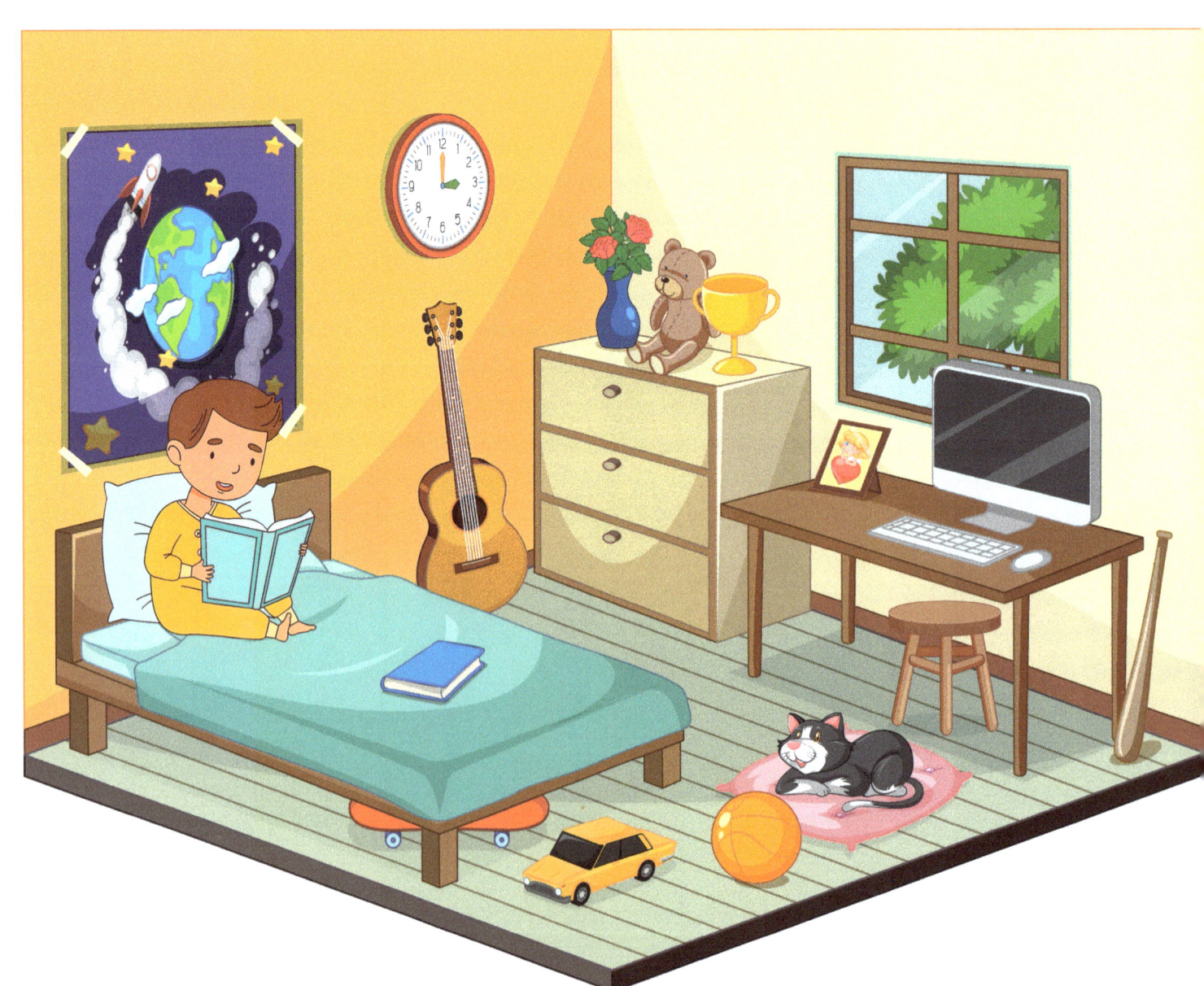

You're in the laugh that sounds like mine.
You're in my hugs, my steps, my spine.

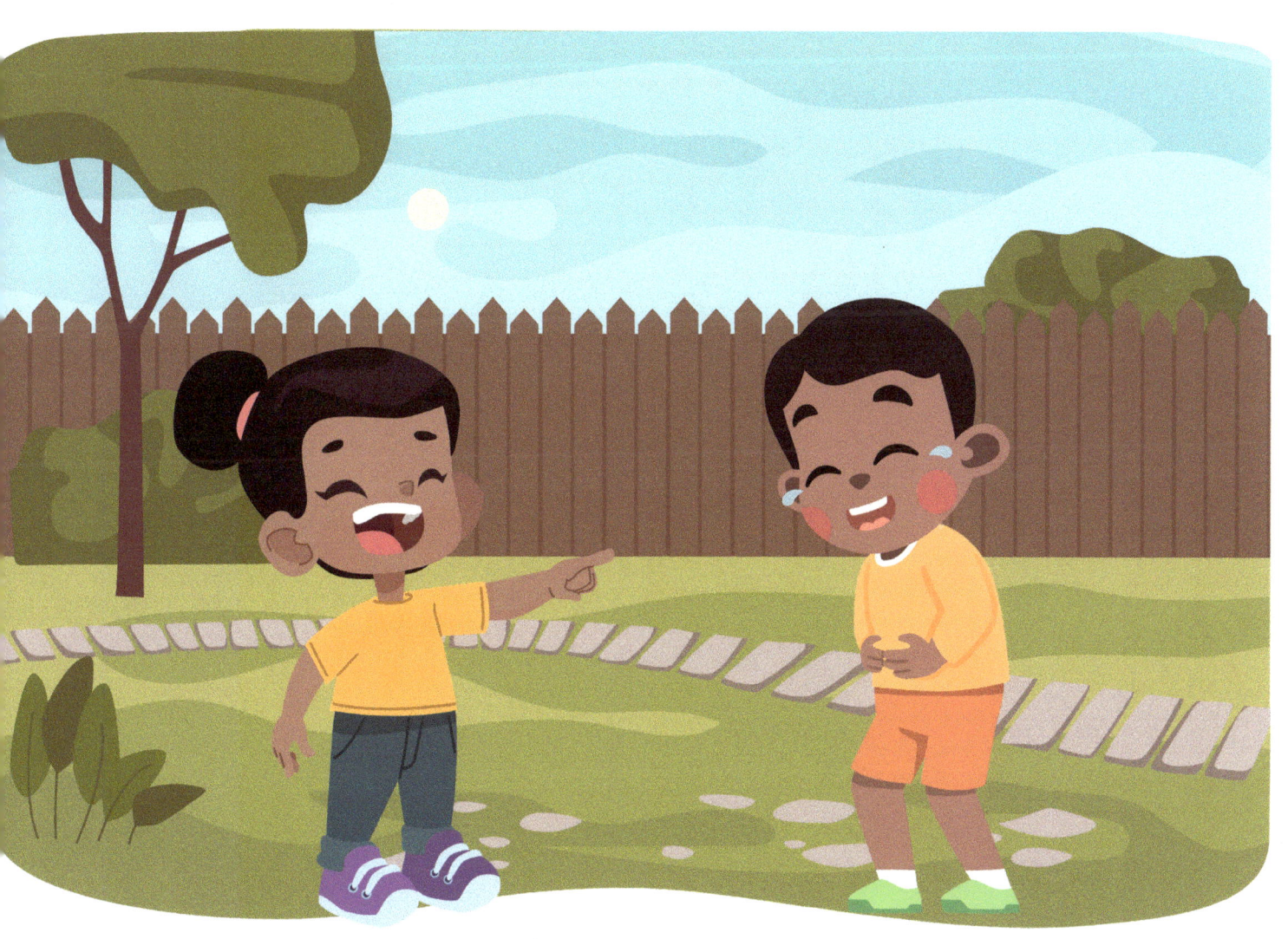

Some days I smile and feel okay.
Some days I cry or walk away.

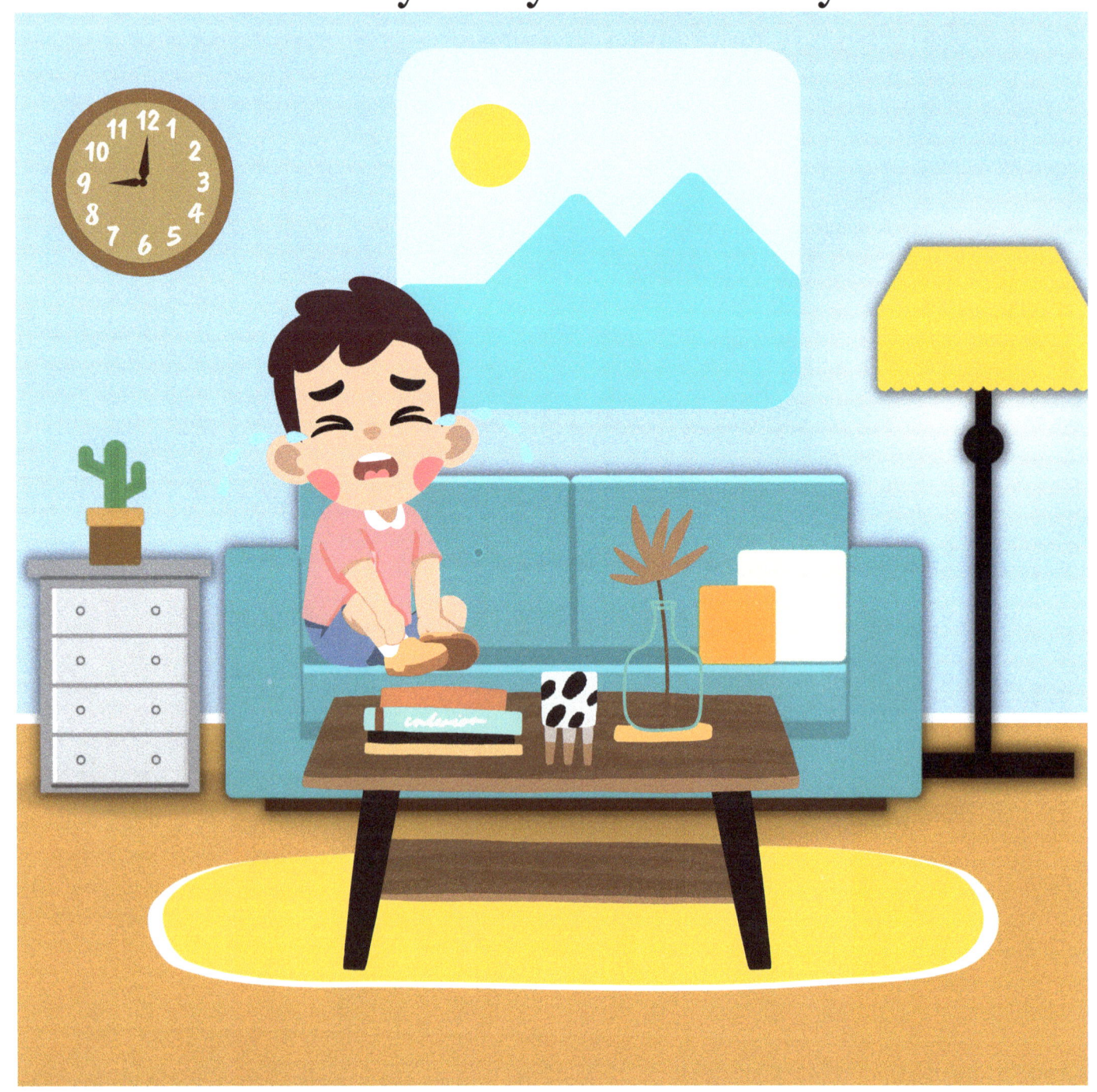

Sometimes I'm mad, and that's alright.
Grief can come in waves at night.

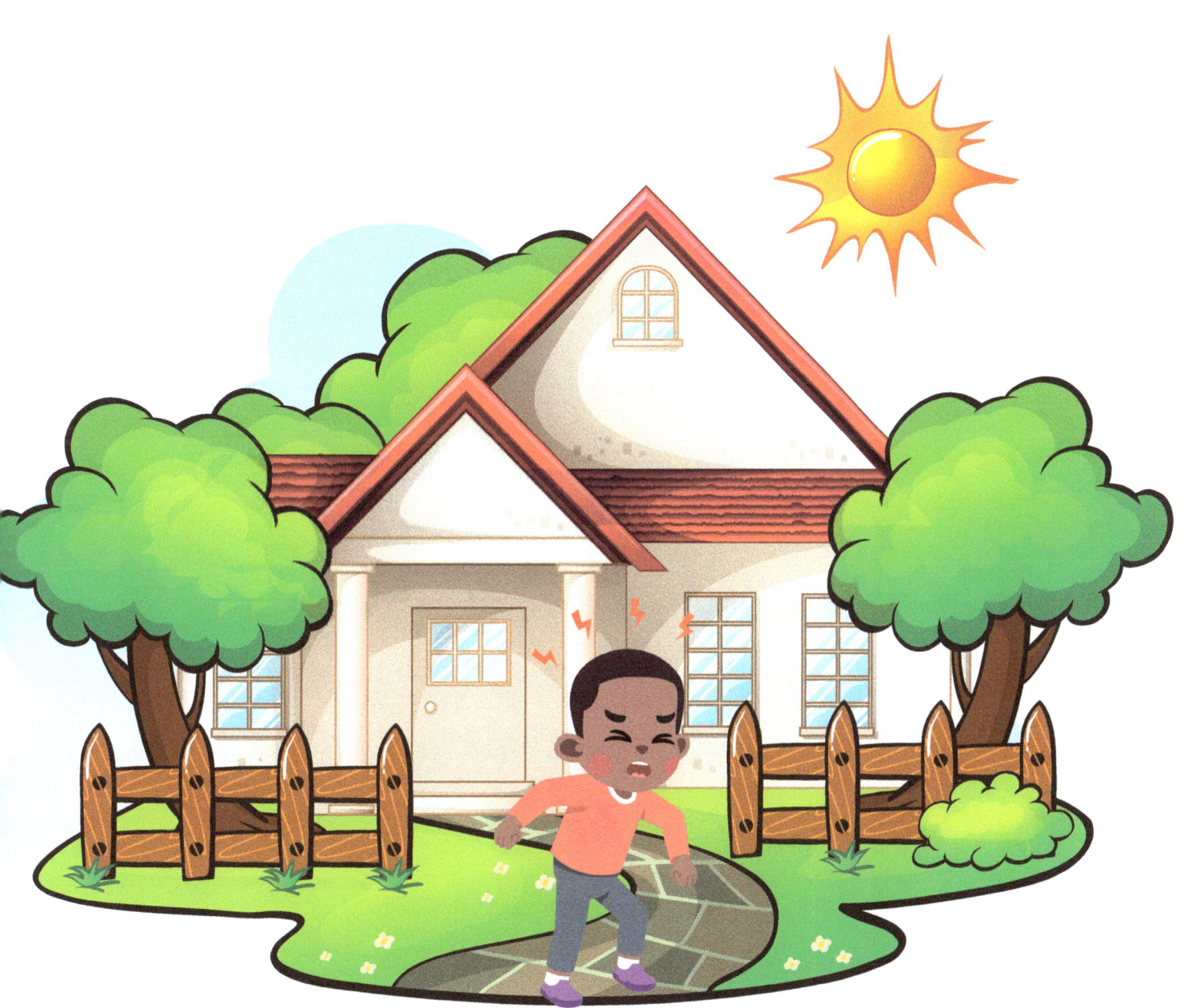

It's okay not to understand.
I still reach out to hold your hand.

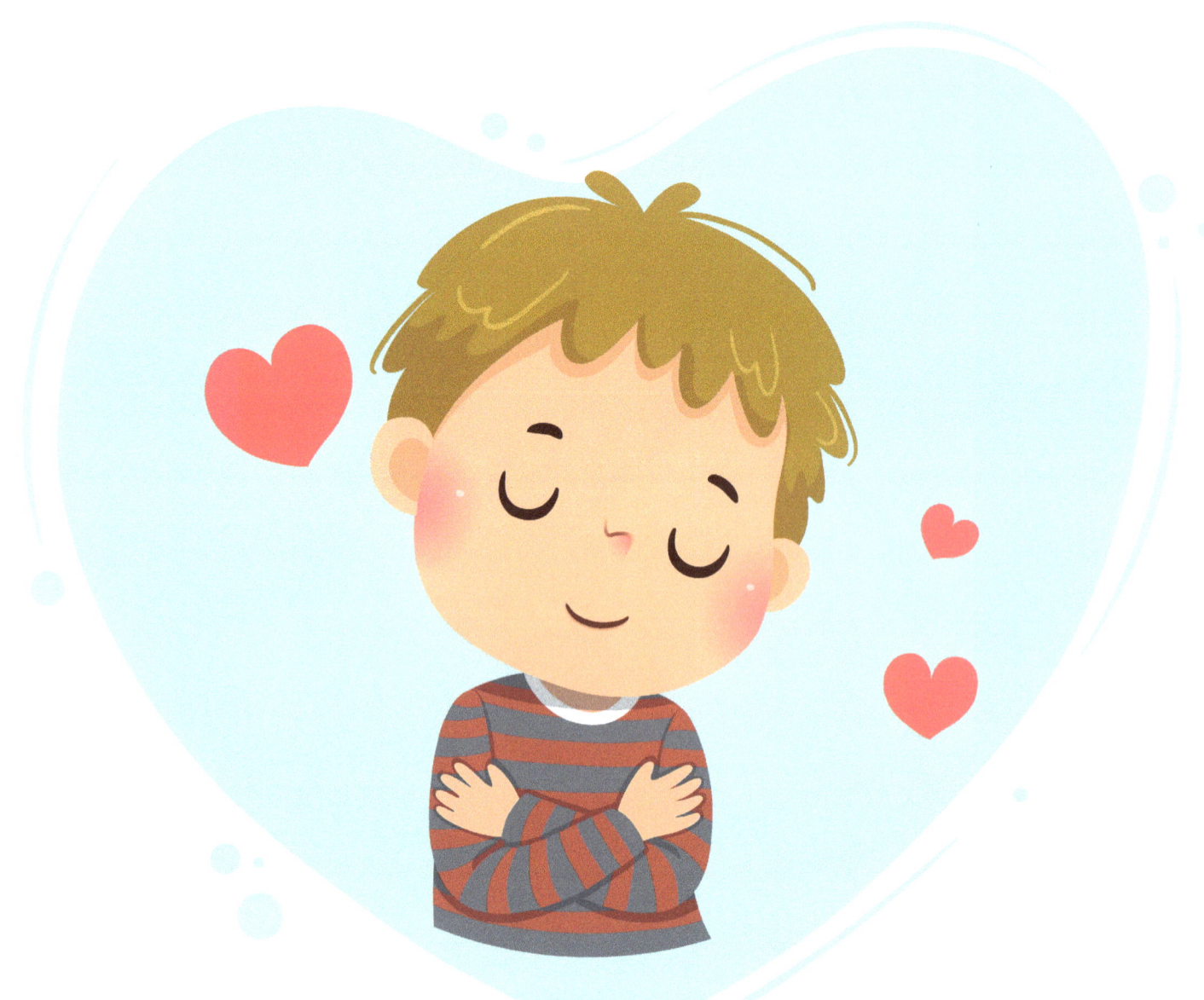

And even though your voice is gone,
I hum your songs and sing along.

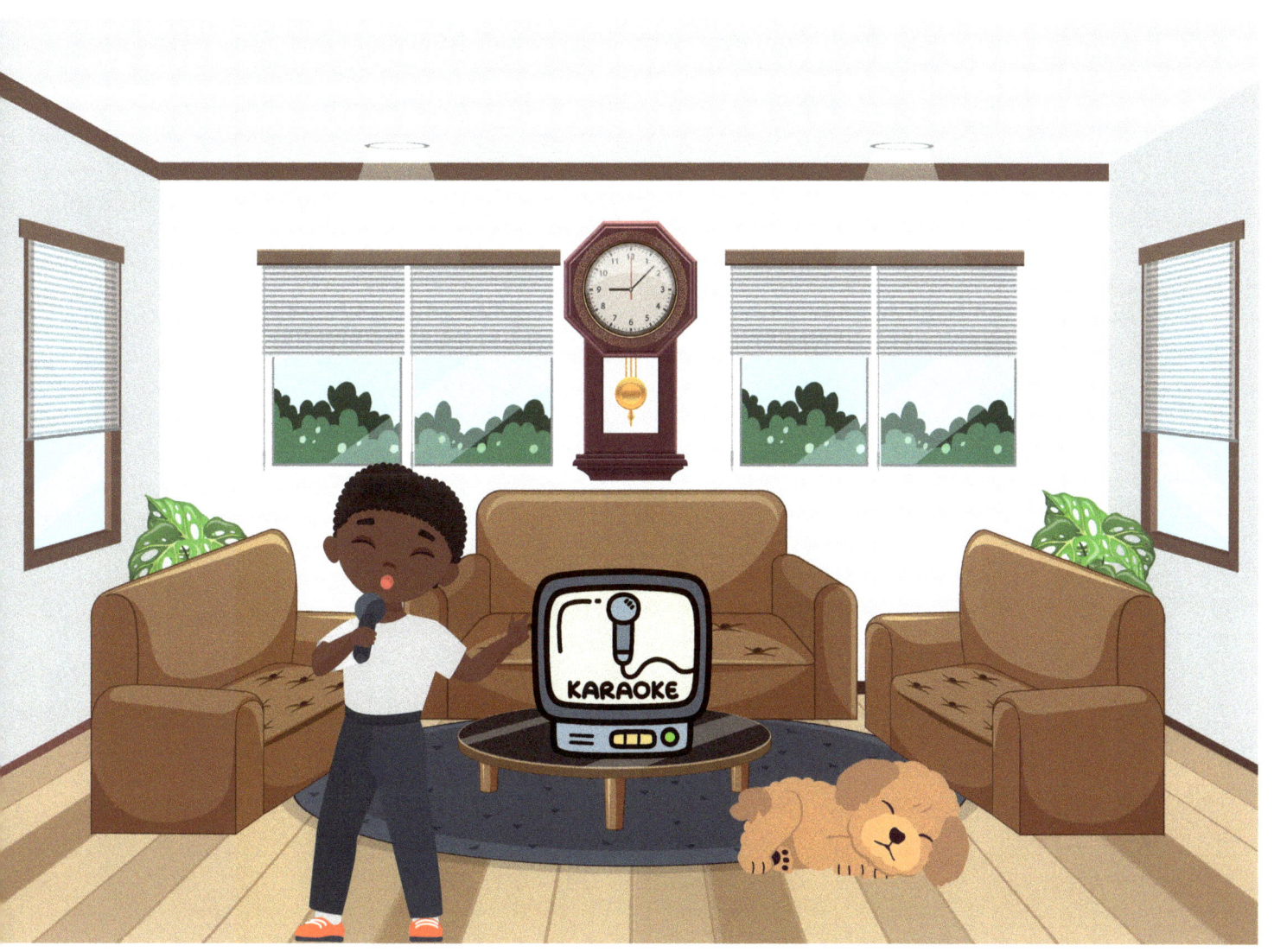

I asked, "Where did you go?" again.
They said, "You're free now, without end."

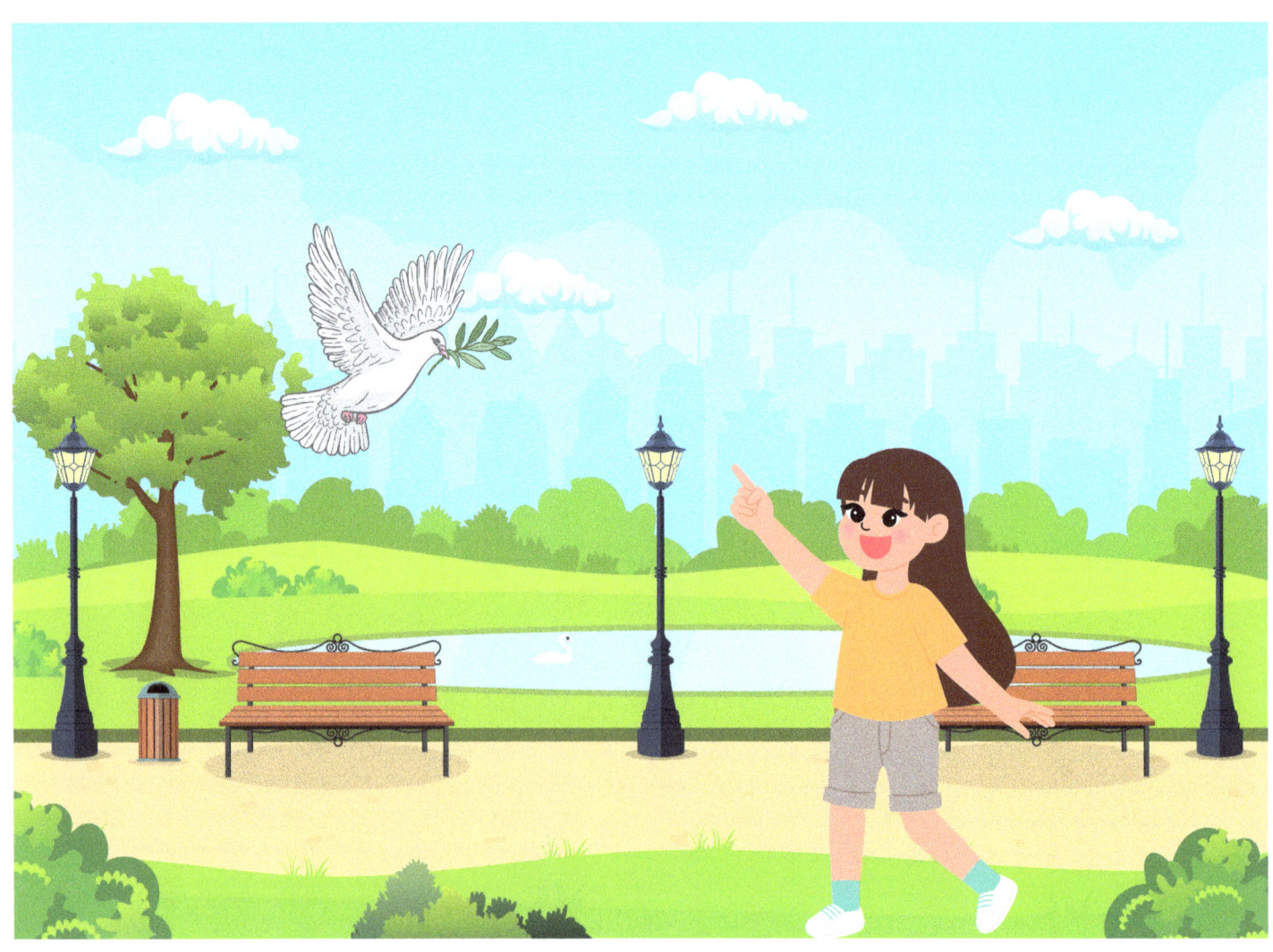

Some say you're stars. Some say the sky.
Some say your soul will never die.

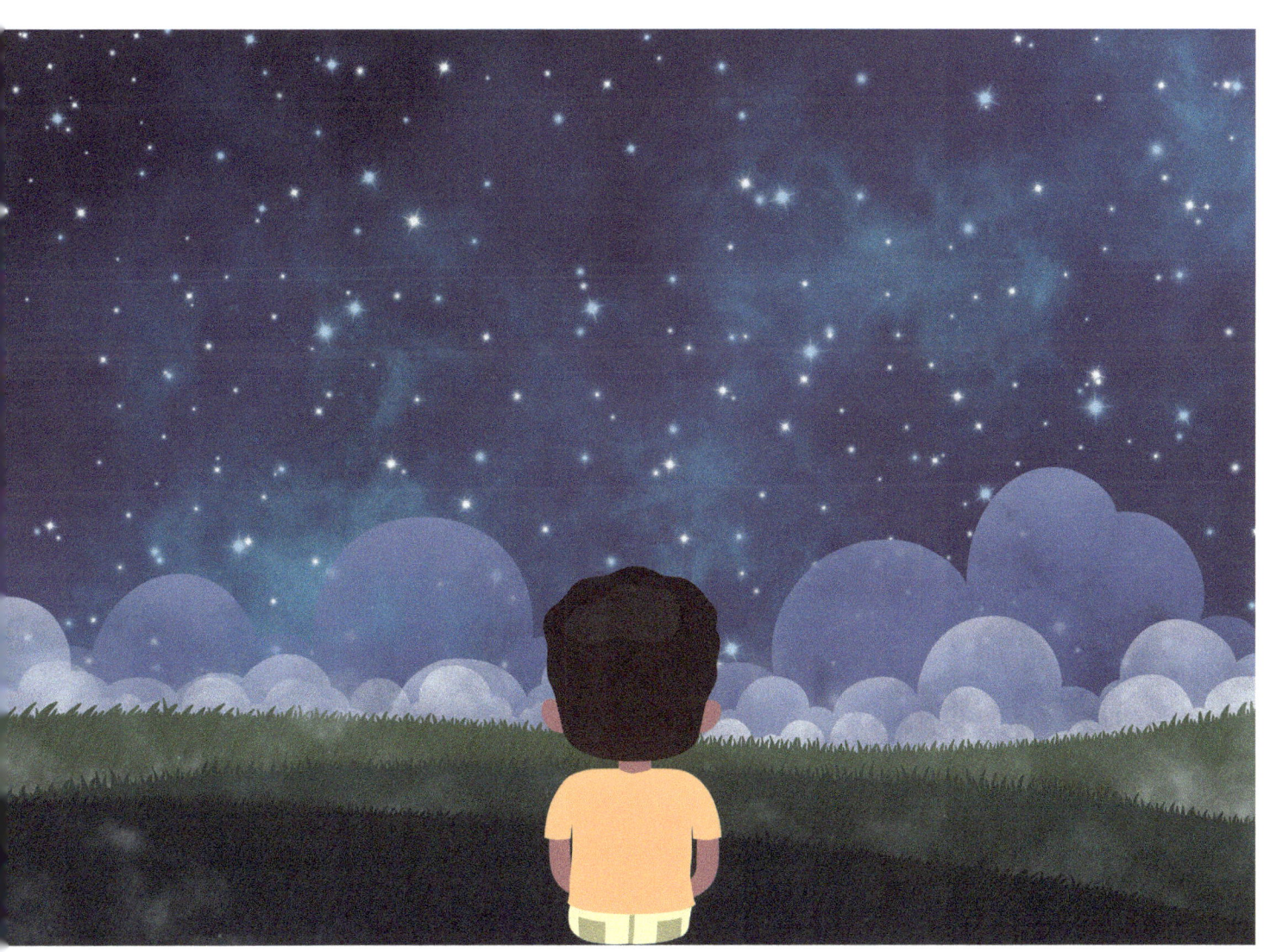

But here is what I truly know:
Love stays, even when you go.

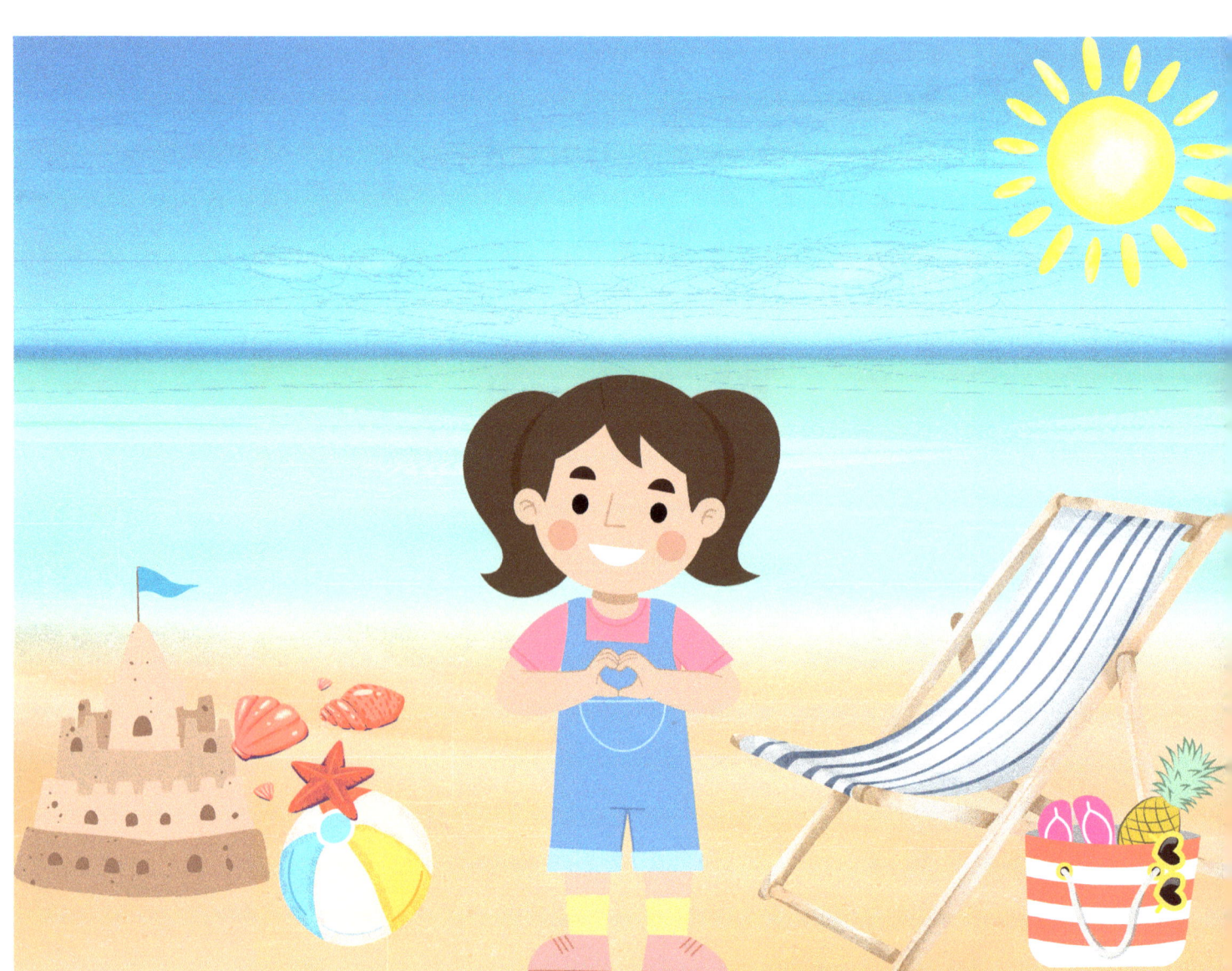

I feel it when the cold winds blow.
You're part of me—from head to toe.

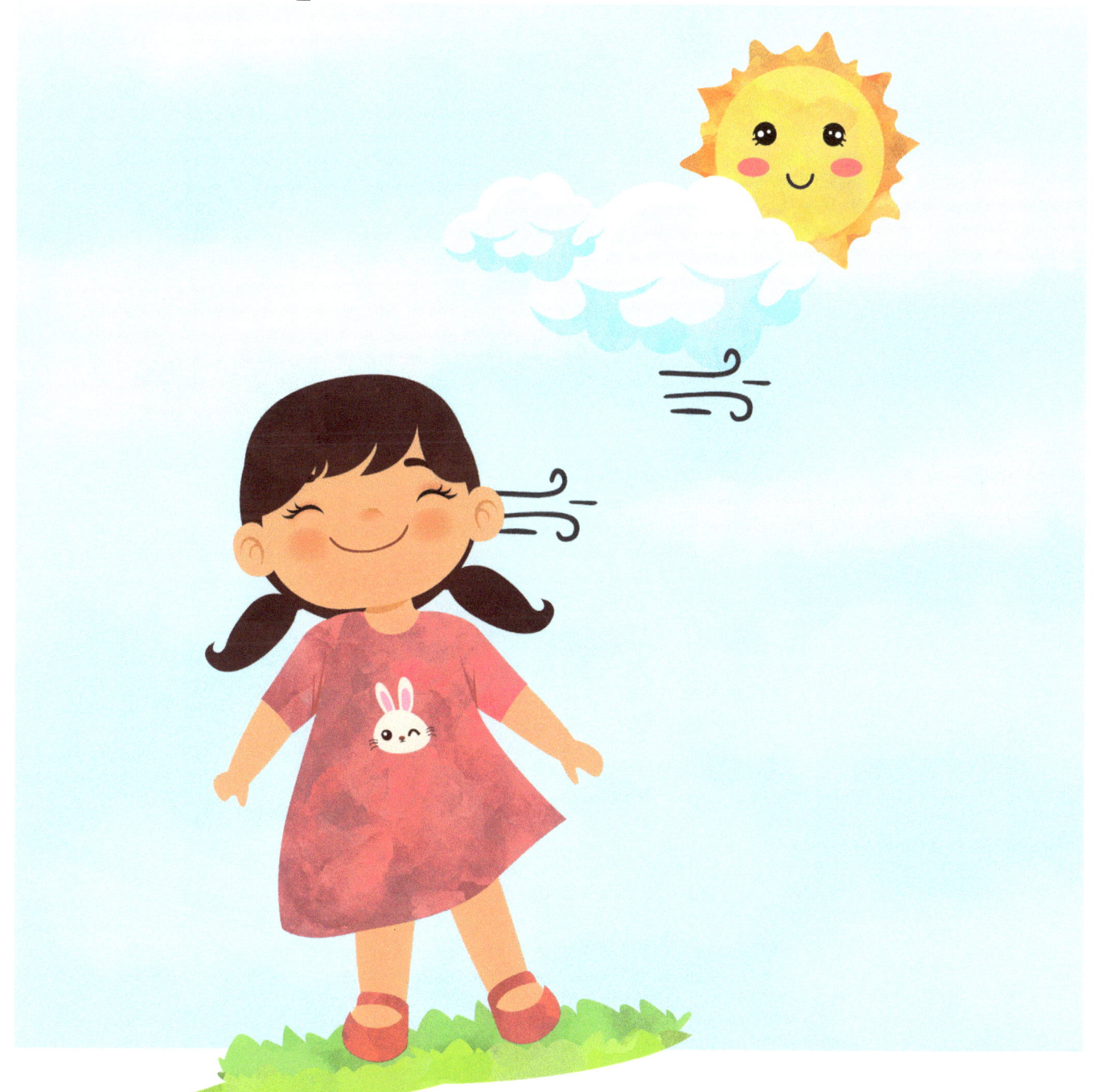

So where you went—I'm not quite sure.
But of one thing, I feel secure:

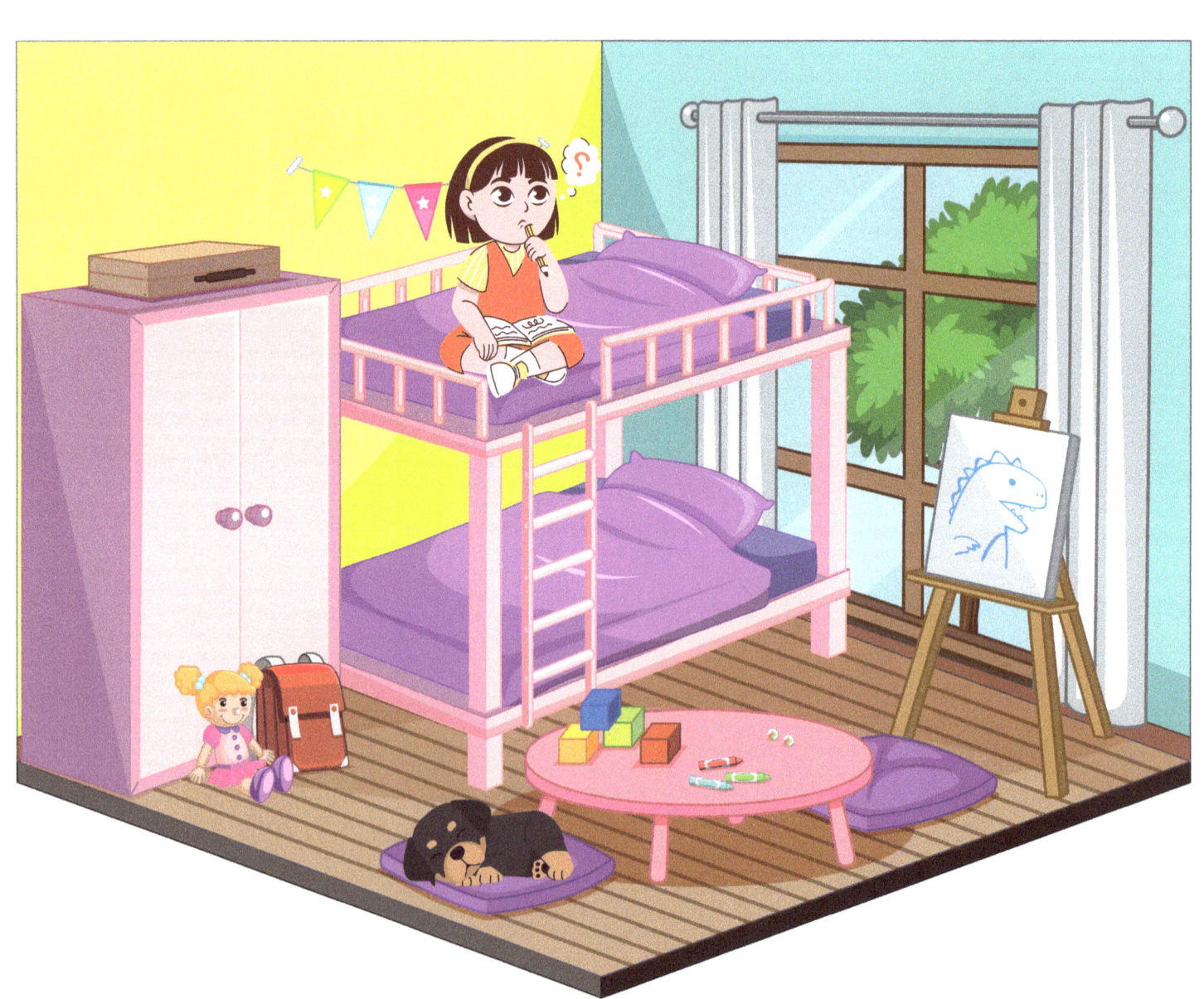

You're in my heart, always with me.
And that's the safest place to be.

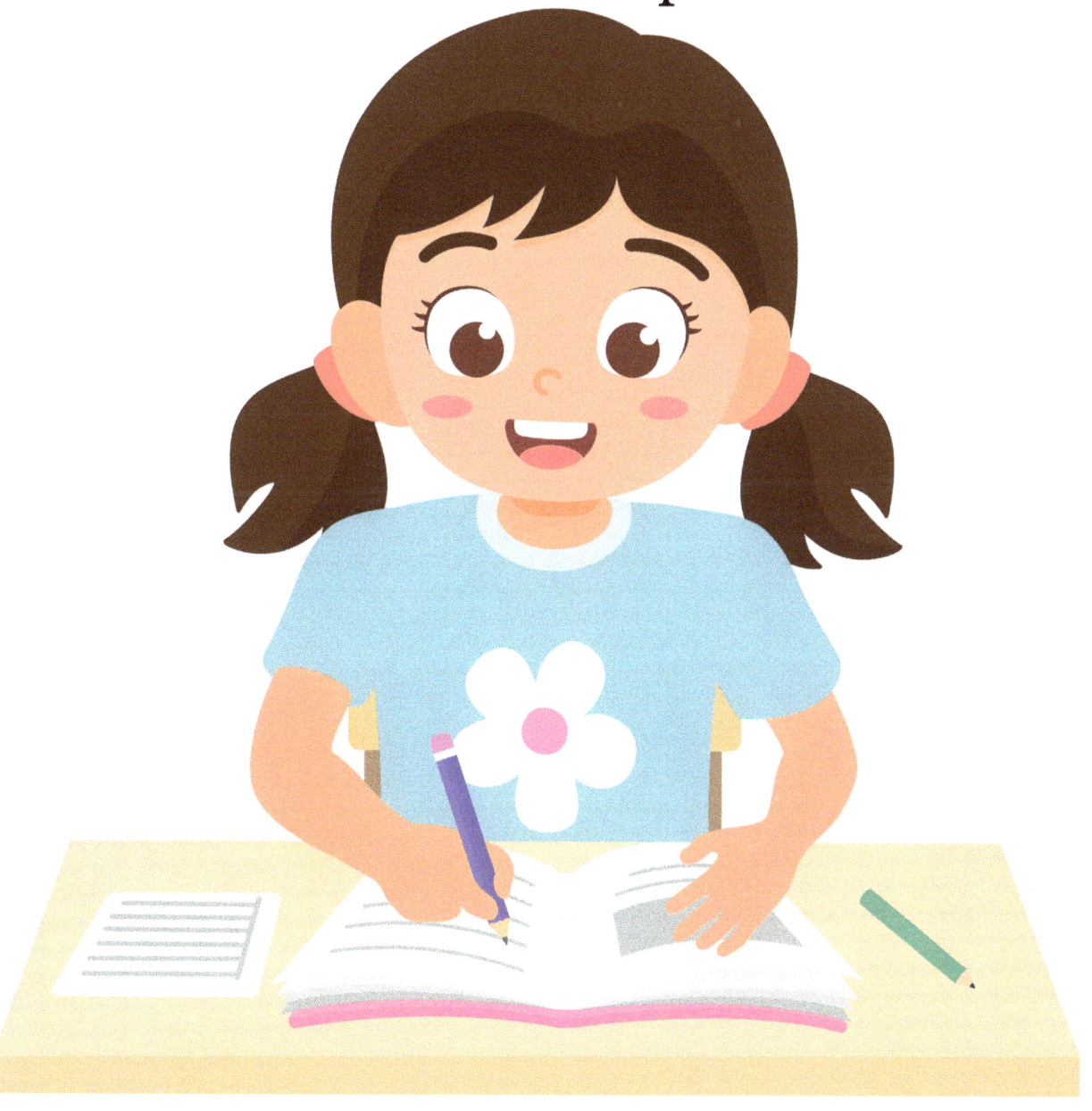

I miss you more than words can say...
But I still talk to you everyday.

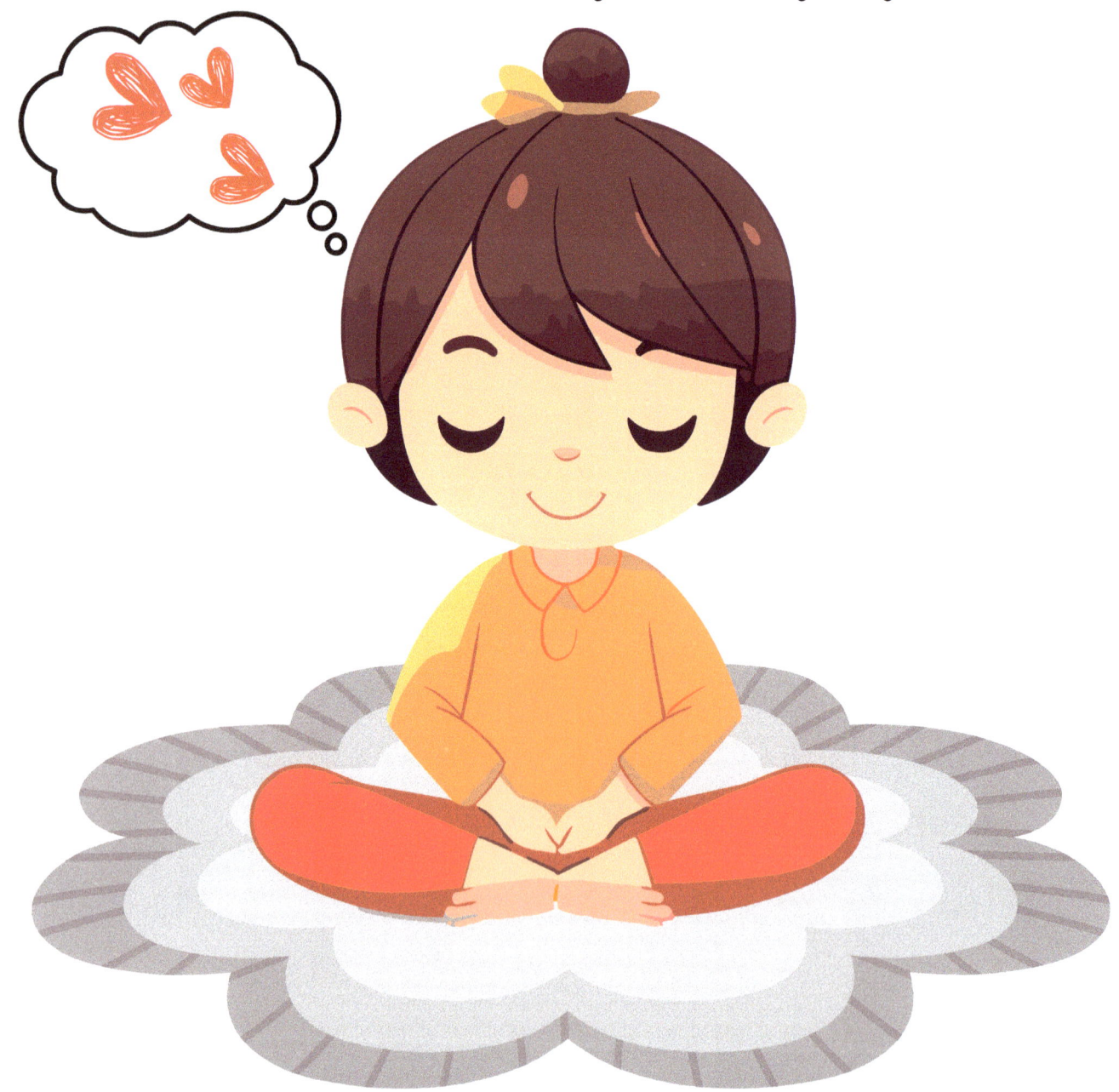

I tell you all the things I do,
And hope somehow you hear me too.

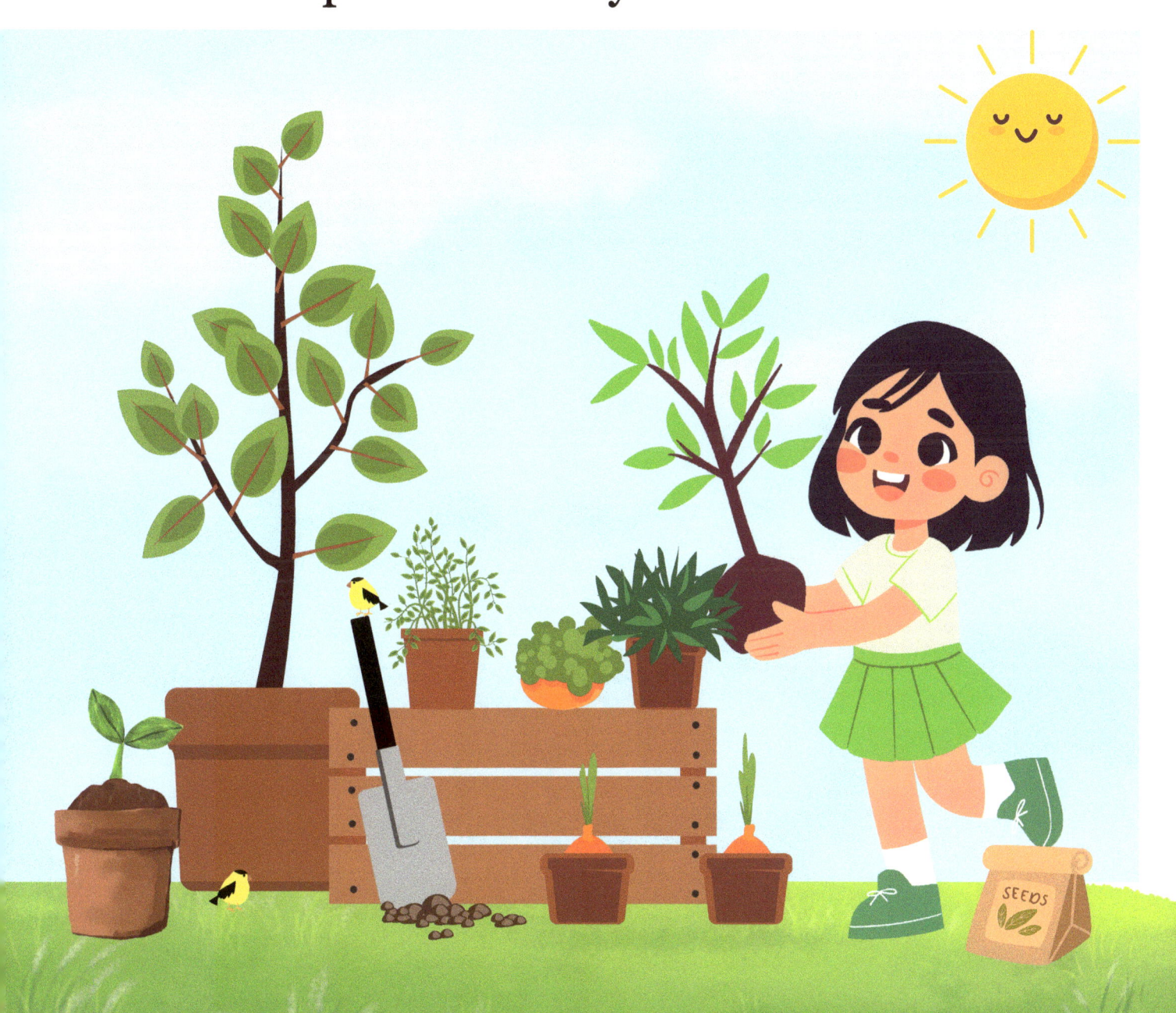

One day I'll see you—maybe so.
But for right now, I'll let you go.

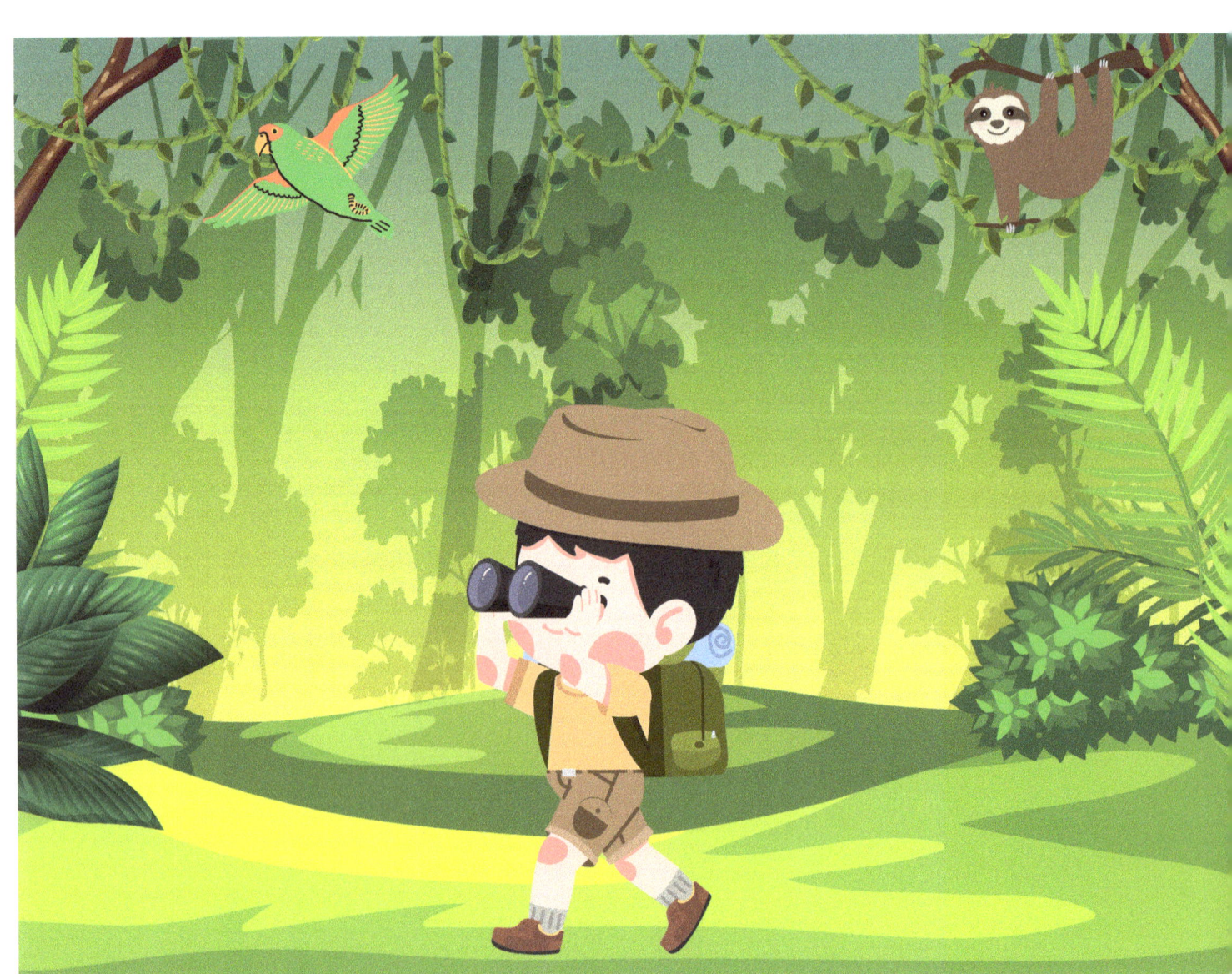

I'll love you big. I'll love you wide.
I'll hold you in my heart inside.

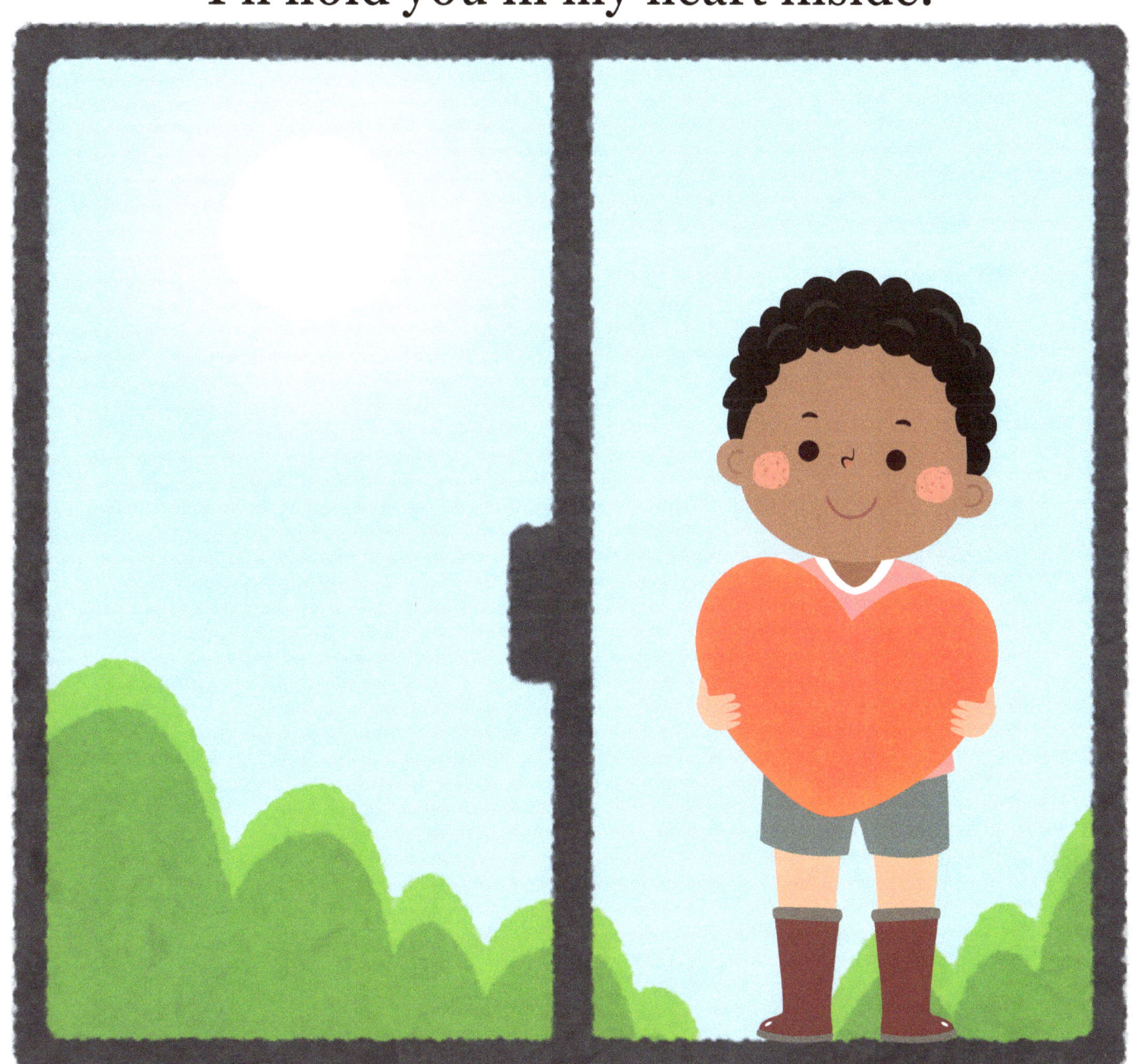

So if you ask, "Where did they go?"
Just know there's more than we can know.

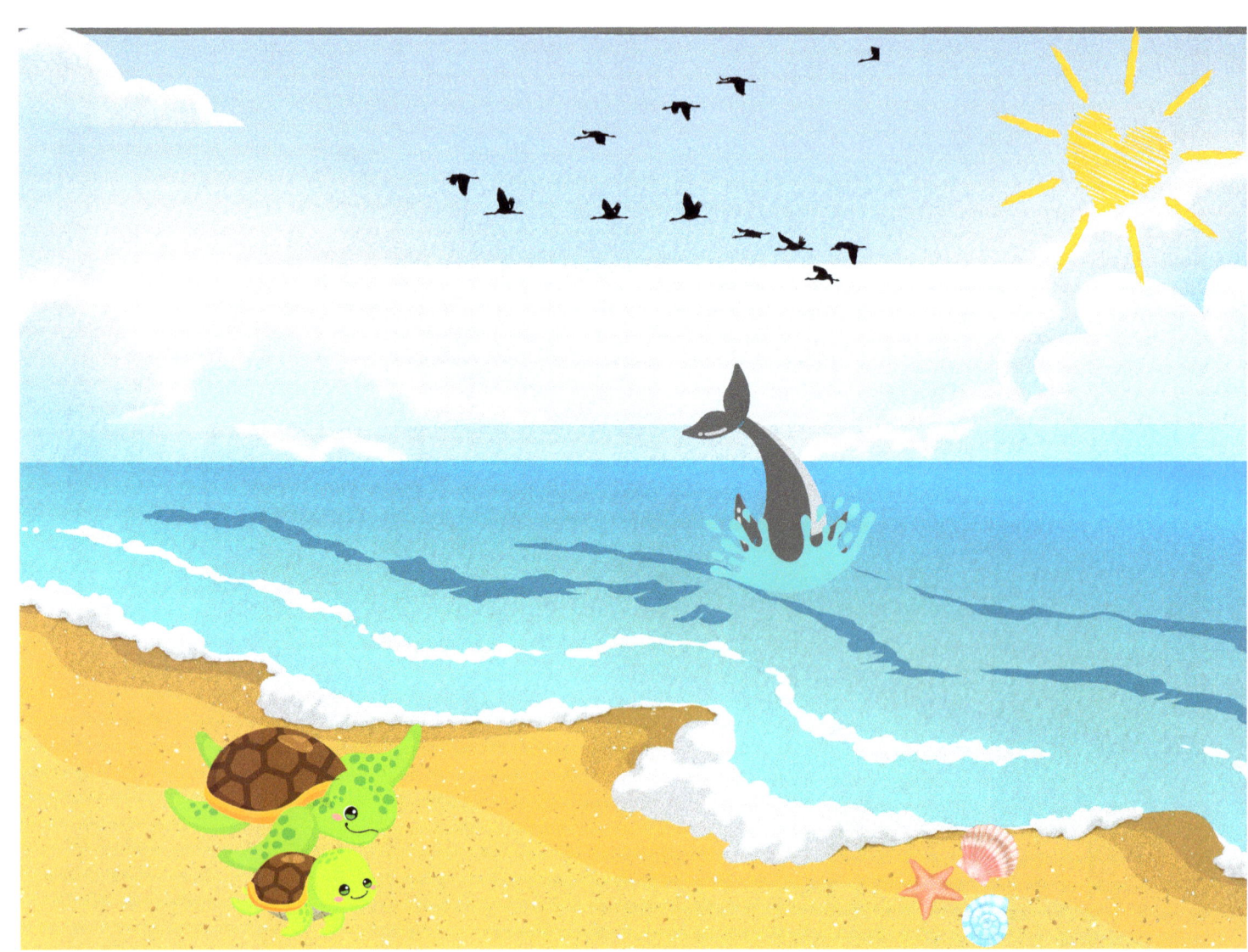

But love, it doesn't end or break—
It's in each breath we ever take.

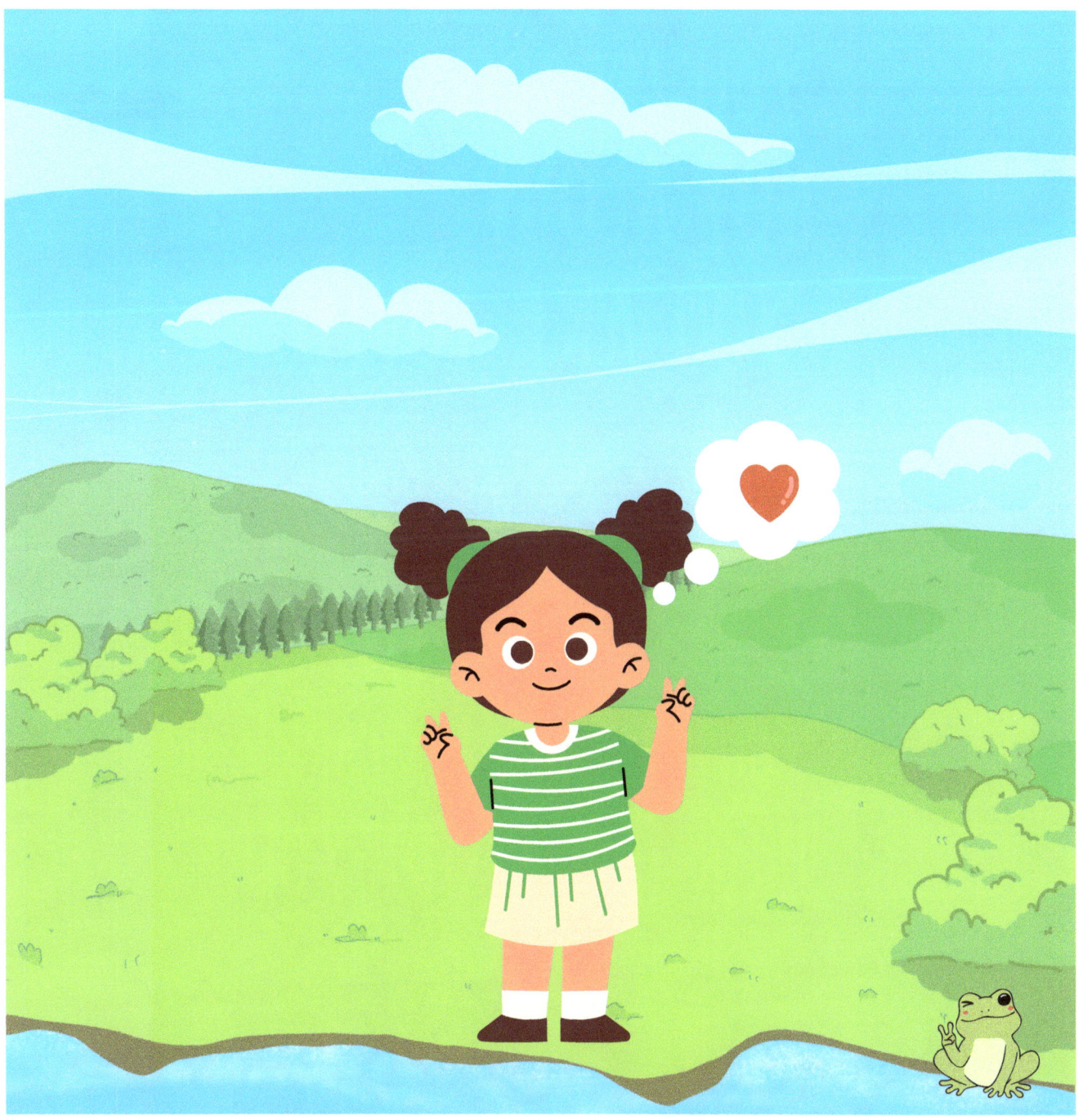

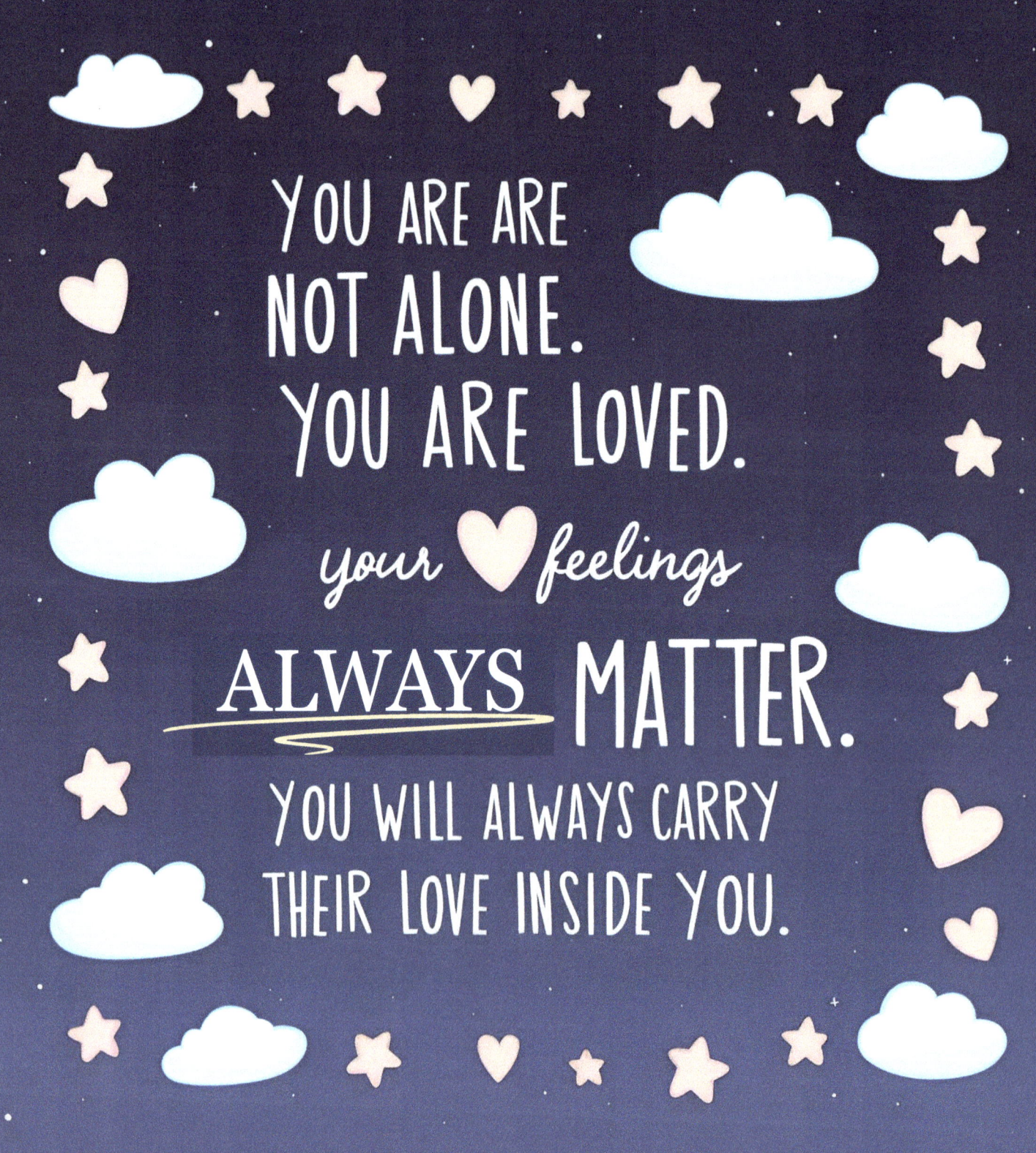

www.ingramcontent.com/pod-product-compliance
Lightning Source LLC
Chambersburg PA
CBHW040002040426
42337CB00032B/5192